AF324713

# A Beginner Guide To Your Air Fryer Toaster Oven Meals

Delicious Air Fryer Toaster Oven Recipes To Stay Fit And Enjoy Your Diet

Eva Morris

## TABLE OF CONTENT

this book has been derived from various sources. Please consult a licensed professional before attempting any techniques outlined in this book.

By reading this document, the reader agrees that under no circumstances is the author responsible for any losses, direct or indirect, which are incurred as a result of the use of information contained within this document, including, but not limited to, — errors, omissions, or inaccuracies.

# Parmesan Cod

Preparation Time: 20 minutes

Cooking Time: 14 minutes

Servings: 4

Ingredients:

- Four cod fillets; boneless
- A drizzle of olive oil
- Three spring onions; chopped.
- 1 cup parmesan
- 4 tbsp. balsamic vinegar
- Salt and black pepper to taste.

Directions:

1. Season fish with salt, pepper, grease with the oil, and coat it in parmesan.
2. Put the fillets in your air fryer's basket and cook at 370°F for 14 minutes. Meanwhile, in a bowl, mix the spring onions with salt, pepper, and the vinegar and whisk
3. Divide the cod between plates, drizzle the spring onions mix all over and serve with a

side salad

Nutrition: Calories: 220; Fat: 12g; Fiber: 2g; Carbs: 5g; Protein: 13g

# Cod And Endives

Preparation Time: 25 minutes

Cooking Time: 30 minutes

Servings: 4

Ingredients:

- Four salmon fillets; boneless
- Two endives; shredded
- 2 tbsp. Olive oil
- ½ tsp. sweet paprika
- Salt and black pepper to the taste

Directions:

In a pan that fits the air fryer, combine the fish with the rest of the ingredients, toss, introduce in the fryer and cook at 350°F for 20 minutes, flipping the fish halfway

Divide between plates and serve right away

Nutrition: Calories: 243; Fat: 13g; Fiber: 3g; Carbs: 6g; Protein: 14g

# Cod And Tomatoes

Preparation Time: 20 minutes

Cooking Time: 15 minutes

Servings: 4

Ingredients:

- 1 cup cherry tomatoes; halved
- Four cod fillets, skinless and boneless
- 2 tbsp. olive oil
- 2 tbsp. Cilantro; chopped.
- Salt and black pepper

Directions:

1. In a baking dish that fits your air fryer, mix all the ingredients, and toss gently.
2. Introduce in your air fryer and cook at 370°F for 15 minutes
3. Divide everything between plates and serve right away.

Nutrition: Calories: 248; Fat: 11g; Fiber: 2g; Carbs: 5g; Protein: 11g

# Spicy Tilapia

Preparation Time: 20 minutes

Cooking Time: 25 minutes

Servings: 4

Ingredients:

- 4 tilapia fillets
- 1/2 tsp. red chili powder
- 1 tsp. garlic, minced
- 3 tbsp. butter, melted
- 1 tbsp. fresh lemon juice
- 2 tsps. fresh parsley, chopped
- 1 lemon, sliced
- Pepper
- Salt

Directions:

1. Line the Baking Pan with foil and set aside.

2. Place fish fillets in the baking pan and season with pepper and salt.

3. Mix together butter, red chili powder, garlic, and lemon juice and pour over fish fillets.

4. Arrange lemon slices on top of fish fillets.

5. Place the baking pan into rack position 2.

6. Set to Convection Bake at 350°F for 15 minutes.

7. Garnish with parsley and serve.

Nutrition:

Calories 149

Fat 12 g

Carbohydrates 4 g

Sugar 0.1 g

Protein 6 g

Cholesterol 38 mg

# Garlic Lime Shrimp

Preparation Time: 20 minutes

Cooking Time: 20 minutes

Servings: 4

Ingredients:

- 1 lb. shrimp, peel and deveined

- 2 tbsps. lime juice

- 2 tbsps. butter, melted

- 1/4 cup fresh cilantro, chopped

- 3 garlic cloves, pressed

Directions:

1. Line the Baking Pan with foil and set aside.

2. Add shrimp into the baking dish.

3. Mix together garlic, lime juice, and butter and pour over shrimp.

4. Toss shrimp well and let it sit for 15 minutes.

5. Place the baking pan into rack position 2.

6. Set to Convection Bake at 375°F for 15 minutes.

7. Garnish with cilantro and serve.

Nutrition:

Calories 195

Fat 7.7 g

Carbohydrates 4.4 g

Sugar 0.4 g

Protein 26.1 g

Cholesterol 254 mg

# Dijon Salmon

Preparation Time: 20 minutes

Cooking Time: 22minutes

Servings: 4

Ingredients:

- 4 salmon fillets
- 1/4 cup Dijon mustard
- 1/4 cup maple syrup
- 2garlic cloves, minced
- 2 tbsp olive oil
- Pepper
- Salt

Directions:

1. Line the Baking Pan with foil and set aside.
2. Place salmon fillets into the baking pan.
3. Mix garlic, olive oil, Dijon mustard, maple syrup, pepper, salt, and pour over salmon. Coat well and let sit for 10 minutes.
4. Place the baking pan into rack position 2.

5. Set to Convection Bake at 400°F for 12 minutes.

6. Serve and enjoy.

Nutrition:

Calories 360

Fat 18 g

Carbohydrates 14 g

Sugar 12 g

Protein 35 g

Cholesterol 78 mg

# Tasty Shrimp Fajitas

Preparation Time: 10 minutes

Cooking Time: 25 minutes

Servings: 4

Ingredients:

- lb. shrimp, peeled and deveined
- 1bell peppers, sliced
- 1 medium onion, sliced
- 1/2 lime juice
- 1 1/2 tbsp. taco seasoning
- 1 1/2 tbsp. olive oil

Directions:

1. Line the Baking Pan with foil and set aside.

2. In a bowl, toss shrimp with remaining ingredients.

3. Spread shrimp mixture on a baking pan.

4. Place the baking pan into rack position 2.

5. Set to Convection Bake at 400°F for 15 minutes.

6. Serve and enjoy.

Nutrition:

Calories 229

Fat 8 g

Carbohydrates 12 g

Sugar 5 g

Protein 27 g

Cholesterol 240 mg

# Parmesan Walnut Salmon

Preparation Time: 10 minutes

Cooking Time: 25 minutes

Servings: 4

Ingredients:

- 4 salmon fillets
- 1/4 cup walnuts
- 1 tsps. olive oil
- 1/4 cup parmesan cheese, grated
- 1 tbsp. lemon rind

Directions:

1. Line the Baking Pan with foil and set aside.

2. Place salmon fillets in the baking pan.

3. Add walnuts into the blender and blend until ground.

4. Mix together walnuts, cheese, oil, and lemon rind and spread on top of salmon fillets.

5. Place the baking pan into rack position 2.

6. Set to Convection Bake at 400°F for 15 minutes.

7. Serve and enjoy.

Nutrition:

Calories 312

Fat 18 g

Carbohydrates 1 g

Sugar 0.2 g

Protein 38 g

Cholesterol 83 mg

# Greek Pesto Salmon

Preparation Time: 10 minutes

Cooking Time: 30 minutes

Servings: 4

Ingredients:

- 4 salmon fillets
- 1/2 cup pesto
- 1/2 cup feta cheese, crumbled
- 2 cups grape tomatoes, halved
- 1 onion, chopped

Directions:

1. Line the Baking Pan with foil and set aside.

2. Place salmon fillet in baking pan and top with tomatoes, onion, pesto, and cheese.

3. Place the baking pan into rack position 2.

4. Set to Convection Bake at 350°F for 20 minutes.

5. Serve and enjoy.

Nutrition:

Calories 447

Fat 28 g

Carbohydrates 8 g

Sugar 6 g

Protein 41 g

Cholesterol 103 mg

# Easy Baked Tilapia

Preparation Time: 10 minutes

Cooking Time: 20 minutes

Servings: 4

Ingredients:

- 1 lb. tilapia fillets
- 2 tbsp. garlic, minced
- 2 tbsp. olive oil
- 2 tbsp. dried parsley
- Pepper
- Salt

Directions:

1. Line the Baking Pan with foil and set aside.

2. Place fish fillets on a baking pan. Drizzle with oil and season with pepper and salt.

3. Sprinkle garlic and parsley over fish fillets.

4. Place the baking pan into rack position 2.

5. Set to Convection Bake at 400°F for 15 minutes.

6. Serve and enjoy.

Nutrition:

Calories 160

Fat 8 g

Carbohydrates 1 g

Sugar 0.1 g

Protein 21 g

Cholesterol 55 mg

# Cajun Catfish Fillets

Preparation Time: 15 minutes

Cooking Time: 20 minutes

Servings: 4

Ingredients:

- 1 lb. catfish fillets, cut ½-inch thick
- 1/2 tsp. ground cumin
- 3/4 tsp. chili powder
- 1 tsp. crushed red pepper
- 2 tsp. onion powder
- 1 tbsps. dried oregano, crushed
- Pepper
- Salt

Directions:

1. Line the Baking Pan with foil and set aside.
2. In a small bowl, mix cumin, chili powder, crushed red pepper, onion powder, oregano, pepper, and salt.

3. Rub fish fillets with the spice mixture on both sides.

4. Place fish fillets in a baking pan.

5. Place the baking pan into rack position 2.

6. Set to Convection Bake at 350°F for 15 minutes.

7. Serve and enjoy.

Nutrition:

Calories 165

Fat 9 g

Carbohydrates 2 g

Sugar 0.6 g

Protein 18 g

Cholesterol 53 mg

# Blackened Mahi Mahi

Preparation Time: 10 minutes

Cooking Time: 17 minutes

Servings: 4

Ingredients:

- 4 Mahi Mahi fillets
- 1 tsp. paprika
- 1 tsp. garlic powder
- 3 tbsps. Olive oil
- 1/2 cayenne
- 1 tsp. oregano
- 1 tsp. cumin
- 1 tsp. onion powder
- 1/2 tsp. pepper
- 1/2 tsp. salt

Directions:

1. Line the Baking Pan with foil and set aside.

2. Place fish fillets on the baking pan and drizzle with oil.

3. In a small bowl, mix together cumin, onion powder, paprika, cayenne, oregano, garlic powder, pepper, and salt.

4. Rub fish fillets with a spice mixture.

5. Place the baking pan into rack position 2.

6. Set to Convection Bake at 450°F for 12 minutes.

7. Serve and enjoy.

Nutrition:

Calories 189

Fat 12 g

Carbohydrates 2 g

Sugar 0.5 g

Protein 19 g

Cholesterol 86 mg

# Salmon Patties

Preparation Time: 20 minutes

Cooking Time: 7 minutes

Servings: 2

Ingredients:

- 1 egg, lightly beaten

- 8 oz. salmon fillet, minced

- 1/4 tsp. garlic powder

- 1/4 tsp. onion powder

- Pepper

- Salt

Directions:

1. Place the air fryer Basket onto the Baking Pan and spray air fryer basket with cooking spray.

2. Add all ingredients into the bowl and mix until just combined.

3. Make small patties from salmon mixture and place onto the air fryer basket.

4. Place assembled baking pan into Rack Position 2.

5. Set to air fry at 400°F for 7 minutes.

6. Serve and enjoy.

Nutritional:

Calories 184

Fat 9 g

Carbohydrates 1 g

Sugar 0.5 g

Protein 25 g

Cholesterol 132 mg

# Crab Cakes

Preparation Time: 20 minutes

Cooking Time: 70 minutes

Servings: 2

Ingredients:

- 1 large egg whites
- 2 green onions, chopped
- 1/2 celery rib, chopped
- 3/4 cup crabmeat, drained
- 1/4 cup breadcrumbs
- 1 1/2 tbsp. mayonnaise
- 1/2 sweet red pepper, chopped
- 1/8 tsp. salt

Directions:

1. Place the air fryer Basket onto the Baking Pan and spray air fryer basket with cooking spray.

2. Place bread crumbs in a shallow dish.

3. In a bowl, add remaining ingredients except for crabmeat and mix well. Gently fold in crabmeat.

4. Drop a tablespoon of crabmeat mixture to the breadcrumbs and slowly coat and shape into patties.

5. Place crab cakes onto the air fryer basket.

6. Place assembled baking pan into Rack Position 2.

7. Set to air fry at 375°F for 12 minutes.

8. Serve and enjoy.

Nutrition:

Calories 151

Fat 4 g

Carbohydrates 21 g

Sugar 5 g

Protein 6 g

Cholesterol 9 mg

# Salmon Dill Patties

Preparation Time: 10 minutes

Cooking Time: 15 minutes

Servings: 2

Ingredients:

- 1 egg

  - 1 tsp. dill weeds

  - 1/2 cup almond flour

  - 14 oz. salmon

  - 1/4 cup onion, diced

Directions:

1. Place the air fryer Basket onto the Baking Pan and spray air fryer basket with cooking spray.

2. Add all ingredients into the bowl and mix well.

3. Make patties from bowl mixture and place onto the air fryer basket.

4. Place assembled baking pan into Rack Position 2.

5. Set to air fry at 375°F for 10 minutes.

6. Serve and enjoy.

Nutrition:

Calories 350

Fat 18 g

Carbohydrates 3 g

Sugar 1 g

Protein 44 g

Cholesterol 172 mg

# Spicy Shrimp

Preparation Time: 10 minutes

Cooking Time: 16 minutes

Servings: 2

Ingredients:

- 1/2 lb. shrimp, peeled and deveined
- 1/2 tsp. old bay seasoning
- 1/2 tsp. cayenne pepper
- 1 tbsp. olive oil
- 1/4 tsp. paprika
- Pinch of salt

Directions:

1. Place the air fryer Basket onto the Baking Pan and spray air fryer basket with cooking spray.

2. Add shrimp and remaining ingredients into the bowl and toss well to coat.

3. Add shrimp into the air fryer basket.

4. Place assembled baking pan into Rack Position 2.

5. Set to air fry at 400°F for 6 minutes.

6. Serve and enjoy.

Nutrition:

Calories 197

Fat 9 g

Carbohydrates 2 g

Sugar 0.1 g

Protein 26 g

Cholesterol 239 mg

# Air Fried White Fish Fillet

Preparation Time: 10 minutes

Cooking Time: 20 minutes

Servings: 2

Ingredients:

- 12 oz. white fish fillets
- 1/2 tsp. lemon pepper seasoning
- 1/2 tsp. garlic powder
- 1/2 tsp. onion powder
- Pepper
- Salt

Directions:

1. Place the air fryer Basket onto the Baking Pan and spray air fryer basket with cooking spray.

2. Spray fish fillets with cooking spray and season with onion powder, lemon pepper seasoning, garlic powder, pepper, and salt.

3. Place parchment paper in the bottom of the air fryer basket.

4. Place fish fillets into the air fryer basket.

5. Place assembled baking pan into Rack Position 2.

6. Set to air fry at 350°F for 10 minutes.

7. Serve and enjoy.

Nutrition:

Calories 298

Fat 13 g

Carbohydrates 1.4 g

Sugar 0.4 g

Protein 42 g

Cholesterol 131 mg

# Mustard-Crusted Sole Fillets

Preparation Time: 5 minutes

Cooking time: 10 minutes

Servings: 4

Ingredients:

- Five teaspoons low-sodium yellow mustard

- One tablespoon freshly squeezed lemon juice

- 4 (3.5-ounce / 99-g) sole fillets

- Two teaspoons olive oil

- ½ teaspoon dried marjoram

- ½ teaspoon dried thyme

- ⅛ teaspoon freshly ground black pepper

- One slice low-sodium whole-wheat bread, crumbled

Directions:

1. Whisk together the mustard and lemon juice in a small bowl until thoroughly mixed and smooth. Spread the mixture evenly over the sole fillets, and then transfer the fillets to the air fry basket.

2. In a separate bowl, combine the olive oil, marjoram, thyme, black pepper, and bread crumbs and stir to mix well. Gently but firmly press the mixture onto the top of fillets, coating them completely.

3. Select Bake, Convection, set temperature to 320ºF (160ºC), and set time to 10 minutes. Select Start to begin preheating.

4. Once preheated, place the basket on the bake position.

5. When cooking is complete, the fish should reach an internal temperature of 145ºF (63ºC) on a meat thermometer. Remove the basket from the oven and serve on a plate.

# Sole And Cauliflower Fritters

Preparation Time: 5 minutes

Cooking time: 24 minutes

Servings: 2

Ingredients:

- ½ pound (227 g) sole fillets
- ½ pound (227 g) mashed cauliflower
- ½ cup red onion, chopped
- One bell pepper, finely chopped
- One egg, beaten
- Two garlic cloves, minced
- Two tablespoons fresh parsley, chopped
- One tablespoon olive oil
- One tablespoon coconut amino
- ½ teaspoon scotch bonnet pepper, minced

- • ½ teaspoon paprika

- • Salt and white pepper, to taste

- • Cooking spray

Directions:

1. Spray the air fry basket with cooking spray. Place the sole fillets in the basket.

2. Select Air Fry, Convection, set temperature to 395ºF (202ºC), and set time to 10 minutes. Select Start to begin preheating.

3. Once preheated, place the basket on the air fry position. Flip the fillets halfway through.

4. When cooking is complete, transfer the fish fillets to a large bowl. Mash the fillets into flakes. Add the remaining ingredients and stir to combine.

5. Make the patties: Scoop out two tablespoons of the fish mixture and shape into a patty about ½ inches thick with your hands. Repeat with the remaining fish mixture. Place the cakes in the air fry

basket.

6. Select Bake, Convection, set temperature
   to 380ºF (193ºC), and set time to 14
   minutes. Select Start to begin preheating.

7. Once preheated, place the basket on the
   bake position. Flip the patties halfway
   through.

8. When cooking is complete, they should be
   golden brown and cooked through. Remove
   the basket from the oven and cool for 5
   minutes before serving.

# Parmesan-Crusted Salmon Patties

Preparation Time: 10 minutes

Cooking time: 13 minutes

Servings: 4

Ingredients:

- 1 pound (454 g) salmon, chopped into ½-inch pieces
- Two tablespoons coconut flour
- Two tablespoons grated Parmesan cheese
- 1½ tablespoons milk
- ½ white onion, peeled and finely chopped
- ½ teaspoon butter, at room temperature
- ½ teaspoon chipotle powder
- ½ teaspoon dried parsley flakes

- $\frac{1}{3}$ teaspoon ground black pepper

- $\frac{1}{3}$ teaspoon smoked cayenne pepper

- One teaspoon acceptable sea salt

Directions:

1. Put all the ingredients for the salmon patties in a bowl and stir to combine well.

2. Scoop out two tablespoons of the salmon mixture and shape into a patty with your palm, about ½ inches thick. Repeat until all the combination is used. Transfer to the refrigerator for about 2 hours until firm.

3. When ready, arrange the salmon patties in the air fry basket.

4. Select Bake, Convection, set temperature to 395ºF (202ºC), and set time to 13

minutes. Select Start to begin preheating.

5. Once preheated, place the basket on the bake position. Flip the patties halfway through the cooking time.

6. When cooking is complete, the patties should be golden brown. Remove from the oven and cool for 5 minutes before serving.

# Cheesy Tuna Patties

Preparation Time: 5 minutes

Cooking time: 17 minutes

Servings: 4

Ingredients:

Tuna Patties:

- 1 pound (454 g) canned tuna, drained
- One egg whisked
- Two tablespoons shallots, minced
- One garlic clove, minced
- 1 cup grated Romano cheese
- Sea salt and ground black pepper, to taste
- One tablespoon sesame oil

Cheese Sauce:

- One tablespoon butter
- 1 cup beer

- • Two tablespoons grated Colby cheese

Directions:

1. Mix the canned tuna, whisked egg, shallots, garlic, cheese, salt, and pepper in a large bowl and stir to incorporate.

2. Divide the tuna mixture into four equal portions and form each piece into a patty with your hands. Refrigerate the patties for 2 hours.

3. When ready, brush both sides of each patty with sesame oil, and then place it in the air fry basket.

4. Select Bake, Convection, set temperature to 360ºF (182ºC), and set time to 14 minutes. Select Start to begin preheating.

5. Once preheated, place the basket on the bake position.  Flip the patties halfway through the cooking time.

6. Meanwhile, melt the butter in a saucepan over medium heat.

7. Pour in the beer and whisk constantly, or until it begins to bubble. Add the grated Colby cheese and mix well. Continue cooking for 3 to 4 minutes or until the cheese melts. Remove from the heat.

8. When cooking is complete, the patties should be lightly browned and cooked through. Remove the cakes from the oven to a plate. Drizzle them with the cheese sauce and serve immediately.

# Chili Tuna Casserole

Preparation Time: 10 minutes

Cooking time: 16 minutes

Servings: 4

Ingredients:

- ½ tablespoon sesame oil

- $\frac{1}{3}$ cup yellow onions, chopped

- ½ bell pepper, deveined and chopped

- 2 cups canned tuna, chopped

- Cooking spray

- Five eggs, beaten

- ½ chili pepper, deveined and finely minced

- 1½ tablespoons sour cream

- $\frac{1}{3}$ teaspoon dried basil

- $\frac{1}{3}$ teaspoon dried oregano

- Acceptable sea salt and ground black pepper, to taste

Directions:

1. Heat the sesame oil in a nonstick skillet over medium heat until it shimmers.

2. Add the onions and bell pepper and sauté for 4 minutes, stirring occasionally, or until tender.

3. Add the canned tuna and keep stirring until the tuna is heated through.

4. Meanwhile, coat a baking dish lightly with cooking spray.

5. Transfer the tuna mixture to the baking dish, along with the beaten eggs, chili pepper, sour cream, basil, and oregano. Stir to combine okay—season with sea salt and black pepper.

6. Select Bake, Convection, set temperature to 325ºF (160ºC), and set time to 12

minutes. Select Start to begin preheating.

7. Once preheated, place the baking dish on the bake position.

8. When cooking is complete, the eggs should be completely set and the top lightly browned. Remove from the oven and serve on a plate.

# Baked Salmon Spring Rolls

Preparation Time: 20minutes

Cooking time: 8 minutes

Servings: 4

Ingredients:

- ½ pound (227 g) salmon fillet
- One teaspoon toasted sesame oil
- One onion, sliced
- One carrot, shredded
- One yellow bell pepper, thinly sliced
- $\frac{1}{3}$ cup chopped fresh flat-leaf parsley
- ¼ cup chopped fresh basil
- Eight rice paper wrappers

Directions:

1. Arrange the salmon in the air fry basket. Drizzle the sesame oil all over the salmon and scatter the onion on top.

2. Select Air Fry, Convection, set temperature to 370ºF (188ºC), and set time to 10 minutes. Select Start to begin preheating.

3. Once preheated, place the basket on the air fry position.

4. Meanwhile, fill a small shallow bowl with warm water. One by one, dip the rice paper wrappers into the water for a few seconds or until moistened, then put them on a work surface.

5. When cooking is complete, the fish should flake apart with a fork. Remove from the oven to a plate.

6. Make the spring rolls: Place ⅛ of the salmon and onion mixture, carrot, bell pepper, parsley, and basil into the rice wrapper's center and fold the sides over the filling. Roll up the wrapper carefully and tightly like you would a burrito.

Repeat with the remaining wrappers and filling.

7.  Transfer the rolls to the air fry basket.

8.  Select Bake, Convection, set temperature to 380ºF (193ºC), and set time to 8 minutes. Select Start to begin preheating.

9.  Once preheated, place the basket on the bake position.

10.  When cooking is complete, the rolls should be crispy and lightly browned. Remove from the oven and cut each roll in half, and serve warm.

# Cinnamon Sweet Potatoes

Preparation Time: 10 minutes

Cooking Time: 30 minutes

Serve: 4

Ingredients:

- Two large sweet potatoes, peel and cut into cubes
- 2 tbsp. brown sugar
- 1/4 cup maple syrup
- 2 tbsp. olive oil
- 1/4 tsp. cinnamon
- **Salt**

Directions:

1. Fit the Cuisinart oven with the rack in position 1.

2. Add sweet potatoes, oil, cinnamon, brown sugar, maple syrup, and salt into the large mixing bowl and toss well.

3. Spread the sweet potatoes in a parchment-lined baking pan.

4.  Set to bake at 400 F for 35 minutes. After 5 minutes, place the baking pan in the preheated oven.

5.  Serve and enjoy.

Nutrition:

Calories 188

Fat 7.1 g

Carbohydrates 31.7 g

Sugar 16.3 g

Protein 0.8 g

Cholesterol 0 mg

# Herb Cheese Sweet Potatoes

Preparation Time: 10 minutes

Cooking Time: 30 minutes

Serve: 6

Ingredients:

- 2 lbs. sweet potatoes, peeled and cut into 1-inch cubes
- 2tbsp olive oil
- 1/4 cup parmesan cheese, grated
- 1tsp dried rosemary
- 1/2 tsp. garlic powder
- **Pepper**
- **Salt**

Directions:

1. Fit the Cuisinart oven with the rack in position 1.

2. Add sweet potatoes into the mixing bowl and oil, rosemary, garlic powder, pepper, salt, and toss well.

3.  In the baking pan, spread sweet potatoes

4.  Set to bake at 425 F for 35 minutes. After 5
    minutes, place the baking pan in the
    preheated oven.

5.  Toss sweet potatoes with parmesan cheese
    and serve.

Nutrition:

Calories 232

Fat 5.8 g

Carbohydrates 42.6 g

Sugar 0.8 g

Protein 3.6 g

Cholesterol 3 mg

# Baked Paprika Sweet Potatoes

Preparation Time: 10 minutes

Cooking Time: 20 minutes

Serve: 4

Ingredients:

- Three sweet potatoes, peel and cut into 1/2-inch pieces
- 2 tbsp. olive oil
- 1/2 tsp. pepper
- 2 tsp. smoked paprika
- 1 tsp. garlic salt

Directions:

1. Fit the Cuisinart oven with the rack in position 1.
2. Add sweet potatoes, paprika, oil, pepper, and salt into the mixing bowl and toss well.
3. Spread the sweet potatoes in the baking pan.

4.  Set to bake at 425 F for 25 minutes. After 5 minutes, place the baking pan in the preheated oven.

5.  Serve and enjoy.

Nutrition:

Calories 155

Fat 7.3 g

Carbohydrates 22.2 g

Sugar 0.7 g

Protein 1.5 g

Cholesterol 0 mg

# Cheesy Broccoli Rice

Preparation Time: 10 minutes

Cooking Time: 20 minutes

Serve: 8

Ingredients:

- 1 1/2 cups cooked brown rice
- One garlic clove, chopped
- 16 oz. frozen broccoli florets
- One large onion, chopped
- 1 tbsp. butter
- 3 tbsp. parmesan cheese, grated
- 10.5 oz. condensed cheddar cheese soup
- 1/3 cup almond milk

Directions:

1. Fit the Cuisinart oven with the rack in position 1.

2. Heat butter in a 10-inch pan over medium heat.

3.  Add onion and cook until tender.

4.  Add garlic and broccoli to the pan and cook until broccoli is tender.

5.  Stir in rice, soup, and milk and cook until hot.

6.  Stir in cheese and pour broccoli mixture into the greased baking dish.

7.  Set to bake at 350 F for 25 minutes. After 5 minutes, place the baking dish in the preheated oven.

8.  Serve and enjoy.

Nutrition:

Calories 244

Fat 8.3 g

Carbohydrates 35.4 g

Sugar 2.7 g

Protein 6 g

Cholesterol 14 mg

# Creamy Broccoli Casserole

Preparation Time: 10 minutes

Cooking Time: 30 minutes

Serve: 6

Ingredients:

- 16 oz. frozen broccoli florets, defrosted and drained

- 1/2 tsp. onion powder

- 10.5 oz. can cream of mushroom soup

- 1 cup cheddar cheese, shredded

- 1/3 cup almond milk

- For topping:

- 1 tbsp. butter, melted

- 1/2 cup cracker crumbs

Directions:

1. Fit the Cuisinart oven with the rack in position 1.

2. Add all ingredients except topping ingredients into the 1.5-qt casserole dish.

3. In a small bowl, mix cracker crumbs and melted butter and sprinkle over the casserole dish mixture.

4. Set to bake at 350 F for 35 minutes. After 5 minutes, place the casserole dish in the preheated oven.

5. Serve and enjoy.

Nutrition:

Calories 203

Fat 13.5 g

Carbohydrates 11.9 g

Sugar 3.6 g

Protein 6.9 g

Cholesterol 26 mg

# Coconut Shrimp

Preparation Time: 10 minutes

Cooking Time: 15 minutes

Serving: 3

Ingredients

- 1 C. almond flour
- 1 C. panko breadcrumbs
- 1 tbsp. coconut flour
- 1 C. unsweetened, dried coconut
- One egg white
- 12 large raw shrimp

Directions:

1. Put shrimp on paper towels to drain.

2. Mix coconut and panko breadcrumbs. Then mix in coconut flour and almond flour in a different bowl.  Set to the side.

3. Dip shrimp into the flour mixture, then into egg white, and then into the coconut mixture.

4. Place into an air fryer basket. Repeat with remaining shrimp.

5. Set temperature to 350°F, and set time to 10 minutes. Turn halfway through the cooking process.

Nutrition: CALORIES: 213; FAT: 8G; PROTEIN: 15G; SUGAR: 3G

# Grilled Salmon

Preparation Time: 10 minutes

Cooking Time: 15 minutes

Serving: 3

Ingredients

- 2 Salmon Fillets
- 1/2 Tsp. Lemon Pepper
- 1/2 Tsp. Garlic Powder
- Salt and Pepper
- 1/3 Cup Soy Sauce
- 1/3 Cup Sugar
- 1 Tbsp. Olive Oil

Directions:

1. Season salmon fillets with lemon pepper, garlic powder, and salt. In a shallow bowl, add a third cup of water and combine the olive oil, soy sauce, and sugar. Place salmon in the bowl and immerse in the sauce. Cover with cling film and allow

marinating in the refrigerator for at least an hour.

2. Preheat the Cuisinart Air Fryer Oven at 350 degrees.

3. Place salmon into the air fryer and cook for 10 minutes or more until the fish is tender.

4. Serve with lemon wedges

# Bacon-Wrapped Shrimp

Preparation Time: 5 minutes

Cooking Time: 10 minutes

Serving: 4

Ingredients:

- 1¼ pound tiger shrimp, peeled and deveined
- 1 pound bacon

Directions:

1. Wrap each shrimp with a slice of bacon.
2. Refrigerate for about 20 minutes.
3. Preheat the Cuisinart Air Fryer Oven to 390 degrees F.
4. Arrange the shrimp in the air fryer basket.
5. Cook for about 5-7 minutes.

# Crispy Paprika Fish Fillets

Preparation Time: 5 minutes

Cooking Time: 15 minutes

Serving: 20

Ingredients:

- 1/2 cup seasoned breadcrumbs
- One tablespoon balsamic vinegar
- 1/2 teaspoon seasoned salt
- One teaspoon paprika
- 1/2 teaspoon ground black pepper
- One teaspoon celery seed
- Two fish fillets halved
- One egg, beaten

Directions:

1. Add the breadcrumbs, vinegar, salt, paprika, ground black pepper, and celery seeds to your food processor—process for about 30 seconds.

2. Coat the fish fillets with the beaten egg; then, coat them with the breadcrumbs

mixture.

3. Pour into the Oven rack/basket. Place the
   Rack on the middle-shelf of the Cuisinart
   Air Fryer Oven. Set temperature to 350°F,
   and set time to 15 minutes.

# Air Fryer Salmon

Preparation Time: 10 minutes

Cooking Time: 15 minutes

Serving: 2

Ingredients

- ½ tsp. Salt
- ½ tsp. Garlic powder
- ½ tsp. smoked paprika
- Salmon

Directions:

1. Mix spices and sprinkle onto salmon.

2. Place seasoned salmon into the Cuisinart Air Fryer Oven.

3. Pour into the Oven rack/basket. Place the Rack on the middle-shelf of the Cuisinart Air Fryer Oven. Set temperature to 400°F, and set time to 10 minutes.

Nutrition: CALORIES: 185; FAT: 11G; PROTEIN: 21G; SUGAR: 0G

# Steamed Salmon & Sauce

Preparation Time: 5minutes

Cooking Time: 10 minutes

Serving: 2

Ingredients

- 1 cup Water

- 2 x 6 oz. Fresh Salmon

- 2 Tsp. Vegetable Oil

- A Pinch of Salt for Each Fish

- ½ cup Plain Greek Yogurt

- ½ cup Sour Cream

- 2 Tbsp. Finely Chopped Dill (Keep a bit for garnishing)

- A Pinch of Salt to Taste

Directions:

1. Pour the water into the Cuisinart Air Fryer Oven tray and start heating to 285° F.

2. Drizzle oil over the fish and spread it. Salt the fish to taste.

3. Now pop it into the Cuisinart Air Fryer Oven
   for 10 min.

4. In the meantime, mix the yogurt, cream,
   dill, and salt to make the sauce. When the
   fish is done, serve with the sauce and
   garnish with sprigs of dill.

# Sweet And Savory Breaded Shrimp

Preparation Time: 5 minutes

Cooking Time: 20 minutes

Serving: 2

Ingredients

- ½ pound of fresh shrimp, peeled from their shells and rinsed

- Two raw eggs

- ½ cup of breadcrumbs (we like Panko, but any brand or home recipe will do)

- ½ white onion, peeled and rinsed and finely chopped

- One teaspoon of ginger-garlic paste

- ½ teaspoon of turmeric powder

- ½ teaspoon of red chili powder

- ½ teaspoon of cumin powder

- ½ teaspoon of black pepper powder

- •        ½ teaspoon of dry mango powder

- •        Pinch of salt

Directions:

1. Cover the air fryer's basket with a lining of tin foil, leaving the edges uncovered to allow air to circulate through the basket.

2. Preheat the Cuisinart Air Fryer Oven to 350 degrees.

3. In a large mixing bowl, beat the eggs until fluffy until the yolks and whites are thoroughly combined.

4. Dunk all the shrimp in the egg mixture, fully submerging.

5. In a separate mixing bowl, combine the bread crumbs with all the dry ingredients until evenly blended.

6. One by one, coat the egg-covered shrimp in the mixed dry ingredients fully covered, and place on the foil- lined air-fryer basket.

7. Set the Cuisinart Air Fryer Oven timer to 20 minutes.

8. Halfway through the cooking time, shake the air fryer's handle so that the breaded shrimp jostles inside and fry-coverage is even.

9. After 20 minutes, when the fryer shuts off, the shrimp will be perfectly cooked, and their breaded crust golden-brown and delicious! Using tongs, remove from the air fryer and set on a serving dish to cool.

# Indian Fish Fingers

Preparation Time: 35 minutes

Cooking Time: 15 minutes

Serving: 4

Ingredients

- 1/2 pound fish fillet
- One tablespoon finely chopped fresh mint leaves or any fresh herbs
- 1/3 cup bread crumbs
- One teaspoon ginger garlic paste or ginger and garlic powders
- One hot green chili finely chopped
- 1/2 teaspoon paprika
- Generous pinch of black pepper
- Salt to taste
- 3/4 tablespoons lemon juice
- 3/4 teaspoons garam masala powder
- 1/3 teaspoon rosemary

- One egg

Directions:

1. Start by removing any skin on the fish, washing, and patting dry. Cut the fish into fingers.

2. In a medium bowl, mix all ingredients except for fish, mint, and bread crumbs. Bury the fingers in the mixture and refrigerate for 30 minutes.

3. Remove from the bowl from the fridge and mix in mint leaves.

4. In a separate bowl, beat the egg; pour bread crumbs into a third bowl. Dip the fingers in the egg bowl, and then toss them in the bread crumbs bowl.

5. Pour into the Oven rack/basket. Place the Rack on the middle-shelf of the Cuisinart Air Fryer Oven. Set temperature to 360°F, and set time to 15 minutes, toss the fingers halfway through.

Nutrition: CALORIES: 187; FAT: 7G; PROTEIN: 11G; FIBER: 1G

# Healthy Fish And Chips

Preparation Time: 5 minutes

Cooking Time: 15minutes

Serving: 3

Ingredients

- Old Bay seasoning

- ½ C. panko breadcrumbs

- One egg

- 2 tbsp. almond flour

- 4-6 ounce tilapia fillets

- Frozen crinkle cut fries

Directions:

1. Add almond flour to one bowl, beat egg in another bowl, and add panko breadcrumbs to the third bowl, mixed with Old Bay seasoning.

2. Dredge tilapia in flour, then egg, and then breadcrumbs.

3. Place coated fish in Cuisinart Air Fryer Oven along with fries.

4. Set temperature to 390°F, and set time to 15 minutes.

Nutrition: CALORIES: 219; FAT: 5G; PROTEIN: 25G; SUGAR: 1G

## Quick Paella

Preparation Time: 7 minutes

Cooking Time: 15 minutes

Serving: 22

Ingredients

- 1 (10-ounce) package frozen cooked rice, thawed
- 1 (6-ounce) jar artichoke hearts, drained and chopped
- ¼ cup vegetable broth
- ½ teaspoon turmeric
- ½ teaspoon dried thyme
- 1 cup frozen cooked small shrimp
- ½ cup frozen baby peas

- One tomato, diced

Directions:

1. In a 6-by-6-by-2-inch pan, combine the rice, artichoke hearts, vegetable broth, turmeric, and thyme, and stir gently.

2. Place in the Cuisinart Air Fryer Oven and bake for 8 to 9 minutes or until the rice is hot. Remove from the air fryer and gently stir in the shrimp, peas, and tomato. Cook for 5 to 8 minutes or until the shrimp and peas are hot, and the paella is bubbling.

Nutrition: CALORIES: 345; FAT: 1G; PROTEIN: 18G; FIBER: 4G

# 3-Ingredient Air Fryer Catfish

Preparation Time: 5 minutes

Cooking Time: 13minutes

Serving: 4

Ingredients

- 1 tbsp. chopped parsley
- 1 tbsp. olive oil
- ¼ C. seasoned fish fry
- Four catfish fillets

Directions:

1. Ensure your Cuisinart Air Fryer Oven is preheated to 400 degrees.
2. Rinse off catfish fillets and pat dry.
3. Add fish fry seasoning to Ziploc baggie, then catfish. Shake the bag and ensure the fish gets well coated.
4. Spray each fillet with olive oil.
5. Add fillets to the air fryer basket.

6. Set temperature to 400°F, and set time to 10 minutes.

7. Cook 10 minutes. Then flip and cook another 2-3 minutes.

Nutrition: CALORIES: 208; FAT: 5G; PROTEIN: 17G; SUGAR: 0.5G

# Tuna Veggie Stir-Fry

Preparation Time: 5 minutes

Cooking Time: 12 minutes

Serving: 4

Ingredients

- One tablespoon olive oil

- One red bell pepper, chopped

- 1 cup green beans, cut into 2-inch pieces

- One onion, sliced

- Two cloves garlic, sliced

- Two tablespoons low-sodium soy sauce

- One tablespoon honey

- ½ pound fresh tuna, cubed

Directions:

1. In a 6-inch metal bowl, combine the olive oil, pepper, green beans, onion, and garlic.

2. Pour into the Oven rack/basket. Place the Rack on the middle-shelf of the Cuisinart Air Fryer Oven. Set temperature to 350°F,

and set time to 4 to 6 minutes, stirring once, until crisp and tender. Add soy sauce, honey, and tuna, and stir. Cook for another 3 to 6 minutes, stirring once until the tuna is cooked as desired. Tuna can be served rare or medium-rare, or you can cook it until well done.

Nutrition: CALORIES: 187; FAT: 8G; PROTEIN: 17G; FIBER: 2G

# Crab Dip

Preparation Time: 18 minutes

Cooking Time: 8 minutes

Servings: 4

Ingredients:

- 8 oz. full-fat cream cheese; softened.
- 2 (6-oz.can lump crabmeat
- ¼ cup chopped pickled jalapeños.
- ¼ cup full-fat sour cream.
- ¼ cup sliced green onion
- ½ cup shredded Cheddar cheese
- ¼ cup full-fat mayonnaise
- 1 tbsp. Lemon juice
- ½ tsp. hot sauce

Directions:

1. Place all Ingredients: into a 4-cup round baking dish and stir until thoroughly

combined. Place dish into the air fryer basket

2. Adjust the temperature to 400 Degrees F and set the timer for 8 minutes. The dip will be bubbling and hot when done. Serve warm.

Nutrition: Calories: 441; Protein: 18g; Fiber: 6g; Fat: 38g; Carbs: 2g

# Sesame Shrimp

Preparation Time: 15 minutes

Cooking Time: 12 minutes

Servings: 4

Ingredients:

- 1 lb. shrimp; peeled and deveined
- 1 tbsp. olive oil
- 1 tbsp. Sesame seeds, toasted
- ½ tsp. Italian seasoning
- A pinch of salt and black pepper

Directions:

1. Take a bowl and mix the shrimp with the rest of the Ingredients: and toss well

2. Put the shrimp in the air fryer's basket, cook at 370°F for 12 minutes, divide into bowls and serve,

Nutrition:

Calories: 199; Fat: 11g; Fiber: 2g; Carbs: 4g; Protein: 11g

# Salmon And Cauliflower Rice

Preparation Time: 30 minutes

Cooking Time: 40 minutes

Servings: 4

Ingredients:

- Four salmon fillets; boneless

- ½ cup chicken stock

- 1 cup cauliflower, riced

- 1 tbsp. butter; melted

- 1 tsp. turmeric powder

- Salt and black pepper to taste.

Directions:

1. In a pan that fits your air fryer, mixes the cauliflower rice with the other Ingredients: except the salmon, and toss

2. Arrange the salmon fillets over the cauliflower rice, put the pan in the fryer, and cook at 360°F for 25 minutes, flipping

the fish after 15 minutes

3. Divide everything between plates and serve

Nutrition:

Calories: 241; Fat: 12g; Fiber: 2g; Carbs: 6g; Protein: 12g

# Tilapia And Salsa

Preparation Time: 20 minutes

Cooking Time:

Servings: 4

Ingredients:

- Four tilapia fillets; boneless
- 12 oz. Canned tomatoes; chopped.
- 2 tbsp. Green onions; chopped.
- 2 tbsp. Sweet red pepper; chopped.
- 1 tbsp. balsamic vinegar
- 1 tbsp. olive oil
- A pinch of salt and black pepper

Directions:

1. Arrange the tilapia in a baking sheet that fits the air fryer and season with salt and pepper.

2. In a bowl, combine all the other ingredients, toss and spread over the fish

3. Introduce the pan in the fryer and cook at 350°F for 15 minutes

4. Divide the mix between plates and serve.

Nutrition:

Calories: 221; Fat: 12g; Fiber: 2g; Carbs: 5g; Protein: 14g

# Garlic Tilapia

Preparation Time: 25 minutes

Cooking Time: 20 minutes

Servings: 4

Ingredients:

- Four tilapia fillets; boneless
- One bunch kale; chopped.
- Two garlic cloves; minced
- 3 tbsp. olive oil
- 1 tsp. Fennel seeds
- ½ tsp. red pepper flakes, crushed
- Salt and black pepper to taste.

Directions:

1. Take a bowl and mix all the Ingredients
2. Put the pan in a fryer, set 360°F, and cook for 20 minutes
3. Divide everything between plates and serve.

Nutrition:

Calories: 240; Fat: 12g; Fiber: 2g; Carbs: 4g; Protein: 12g

# Trout And Mint

Preparation Time: 21 minutes

Cooking Time: 8 minutes

Servings: 4

Ingredients:

- One avocado, peeled, pitted, and roughly chopped.
- Four rainbow trout
- 1/3 pine nuts
- One cup olive oil+ 3 tbsp.
- One cup parsley; chopped.
- Three garlic cloves; minced
- ½ cup mint; chopped.
- Zest of 1 lemon
- Juice of 1 lemon
- A pinch of salt and black pepper

Directions:

1. Pat dry the trout, season with salt and pepper, and rub with 3 tbsp. oil

2. Put the fish in your air fryer's basket and cook for 8 minutes on each side. Divide the fish between plates and drizzle half of the lemon juice all over

3. In a blender, combine the rest of the oil with the remaining lemon juice, parsley, garlic, mint, lemon zest, pine nuts, and the avocado and pulse well. Spread this over the trout and serve.

Nutrition:

Calories: 240; Fat: 12g; Fiber: 4g; Carbs: 6g; Protein: 9g

# Salmon And Coconut Sauce

Preparation Time: 25 minutes

Cooking Time:  20 minutes

Servings: 4

Ingredients:

- Four salmon fillets; boneless
- 1/3 cup heavy cream
- ¼ cup lime juice
- ½ cup coconut; shredded
- ¼ cup coconut cream
- 1 tsp. lime zest; grated
- A pinch of salt and black pepper

Directions:

1. Take a bowl and mix all the Ingredients: except the salmon and whisk.

2. Arrange the fish in a pan that fits your air fryer, drizzle the coconut sauce all over, put the pan in the machine, and cook at 360°F for 20 minutes

3.  Divide between plates and serve

Nutrition:

Calories: 227; Fat: 12g; Fiber: 2g; Carbs: 4g; Protein: 9g

# Simple Salmon

Preparation Time: 22 minutes

Cooking Time: 15 minutes

Servings: 2

Ingredients:

- 2 (4-oz.salmon fillets, skin removed
- One medium lemon.
- 2 tbsp. unsalted butter; melted.
- ½ tsp. Dried dill
- ½ tsp. Garlic powder.

Directions:

1. Place each fillet on a 5" × 5" square of aluminum foil. Drizzle with butter and sprinkle with garlic powder.

2. Zest half of the lemon and sprinkle zest over salmon. Slice the other half of the lemon and lay two slices on each piece of salmon. Sprinkle dill over salmon

3. Gather and fold foil at the top and sides to fully close packets. Place foil packets into the air fryer basket. Adjust the

temperature to 400 Degrees F and set the timer for 12 minutes

4. Salmon will be easily flaked and have an internal temperature of at least 145 Degrees F when fully cooked.

Nutrition:

Calories: 252; Protein: 29g; Fiber: 4g; Fat: 15g; Carbs: 2g

# Cajun Salmon

Preparation Time: 12 minutes

Cooking Time: 8 minutes

Servings: 2

Ingredients:

- 2 (4-oz.salmon fillets, skin removed
- 2 tbsp. Unsalted butter; melted.
- 1 tsp. Paprika
- ¼ tsp. Ground black pepper
- ⅛ tsp. Ground cayenne pepper
- ½ tsp. Garlic powder.

Directions:

1. Brush each fillet with butter. Combine remaining ingredients: in a small bowl and then rub onto fish. Place fillets into the air fryer basket

2. Adjust the temperature to 390 Degrees F and set the timer for 7 minutes. When fully cooked, the internal temperature will be 145 Degrees F. Serve immediately.

Nutrition:

Calories: 253; Protein: 29g; Fiber: 4g; Fat: 16g; Carbs: 4g

# Salmon And Sauce

Preparation Time: 25 minutes

Cooking Time: 20 minutes

Servings: 4

Ingredients:

- Four salmon fillets; boneless

- Two garlic cloves; minced

- ¼ cup ghee; melted

- ½ cup heavy cream

- 1 tbsp. Chives; chopped.

- 1 tsp. lemon juice

- 1 tsp. Dill; chopped.

- A pinch of salt and black pepper

Directions:

1. Take a bowl and mix all the Ingredients: except the salmon, and whisk well.

2. Arrange the salmon in a pan that fits the air fryer, drizzle the sauce all over, introduce the pan in the machine, and cook at 360°F for 20 minutes. Divide everything

between plates and serve

Nutrition: Calories: 220; Fat: 14g; Fiber: 2g; Carbs: 5g; Protein: 12g

CPSIA information can be obtained
at www.ICGtesting.com
Printed in the USA
BVHW051858130721
611835BV00002B/208